WHAT PEOPLE WORKING WI

Ruth is very knowledgeable and passionate about this subject, has her own experience, provided lots of helpful information and resource directions.

Example from a series of workshops run for the
Royal College of Midwives

The workshop was highly appreciated by staff. The content was extremely informative and it was very useful to have guidance from such an expert source – especially as reliable advice on the menopause is frustratingly difficult to access, even for those who think to look for it. Ruth takes a balanced approach and everything is backed up by medical evidence. During the session she creates a relaxed atmosphere in which it is easy to voice concerns and ask any type of question. I would strongly recommend this workshop not just to those experiencing symptoms of the menopause, but also for younger women who deserve to be better informed and prepared to make the right choices at the best time for them.

GDST (The Girls' Day School Trust)

'Ruth covered what can be an embarrassing topic in a really professional and fun manner... would recommend this course to others.'

'Fabulously detailed without being overwhelming... you didn't mind us interrupting!'

'Excellent, great sincerity and understanding from Ruth... learnt things I never knew.'

'Would recommend course to others, very informative... and at an appropriate level... excellent course, learned a lot.'

'Ruth... you were a real catalyst and eye opener and even better still, you made it OK and relevant for a group of friends to actually discuss the details of how we were feeling, rather than just having general moans. We have all fed off each other to greater or lesser degrees since the workshop. I can only speak for myself, but I feel empowered since I started unpicking the blocks that form my "symptoms" and one by one I'm trying to practically tackle them.'

'Thank you so much for a very entertaining and informative evening.'

'Excellent information, well explained and easy to grasp, all very well discussed.'

Fabulous, very helpful... if you're thinking about it, stop thinking and just go – and tell all your friends.
The Let's Talk Menopause workshop was very much appreciated by staff. Ruth is extremely knowledgeable and has a great practical approach which puts everyone at ease really quickly. There are still many myths around

the menopause and Ruth manages to dispel the myths and can back up her advice and guidance with medical evidence and a great sense of humour! As a result of positive feedback from staff attending the workshop, we now plan to roll this workshop out to other regions within our organisation.

Historic Environmental Scotland

'Ruth's style immediately put people at ease with her amazing warmth, her humour and infectious laugh, and even the lovely location which was thoughtfully laid out, and had tea and cake.... Often, the really intimate things are avoided in articles and even between women it can be hard to work out how to talk about it. Not with Ruth – she was straight talking, and to the point, and also was very good at making sure that everyone was at ease, as none of us knew each other. She talked to us, ran a question and answer session, which was very well organised, and backed up her talk with very informative notes, along with websites for more research. She helped me immensely, and managed to make sure that the myth busting happened and helped us all understand how thinking had changed. It made me realise just how out of date my GP had been with her advice. It also helps just to be encouraged to share symptoms, and to be told you are not going mad.'

'I have used the websites, and have recommended Ruth's workshops to others, as the time to learn about it is before it starts – forewarned is forearmed.'

All The best

[signature]

MEN...
LET'S TALK
MENOPAUSE

Ruth Devlin

First published in Great Britain by Practical Inspiration Publishing, 2019

ISBN 978-1-78860-080-4

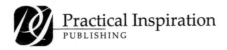 Practical Inspiration
PUBLISHING

TABLE OF CONTENTS

Preface ix

Introduction 1

1. Some basic facts 5

2. The physical symptoms 13

3. The psychological symptoms 29

4. The genitourinary symptoms
    (reproductive and urinary) 35

5. Rare and possible long-term symptoms 41

6. Lifestyle, diet and exercise 45

7. Hormone replacement therapy (HRT) 55

8. Alternative remedies and therapies 65

Postscript… a final few words 73

Useful links and reading 75

PREFACE

Why I wrote this book...

I wrote this book to help men understand this phase of their partner's life. A constant comment when running workshops being... I wish my husband/partner could hear all this information. Would you get a group of men to attend an evening about the menopause? Probably not... so I thought a small compact guide would be useful! I've tried to pack in as much helpful information as possible with good signposting for further information. The good thing is, your partner will find this book useful too!

Before I started to write this guide, I asked several female friends to tell me one thing they thought their husbands or partners would like to know about the menopause.

Being a humorous lot, their replies varied from "Can you get a wife on sale or return?" to the predictable one, "When will I get my sex life back?!"

Then I contacted a large selection of male friends and relatives whose opinions I knew would be honest and, in some cases, blunt. I was surprised, first, by the speed with which the responses came back and, second, by the quality of the responses. Some were predictable, others enlightening; many were insightful. Most of them realised something was going on, but weren't sure what, and felt at a loss as to how to cope or help in any way. All said they would like more information and would appreciate "an idiot's guide to the menopause", but pleaded, "Don't make it too long, we just want facts and no fluffy bits, but add a few hyperlinks." So here you are!

Before I begin... as I'm not sure if I'm referring to your wife, partner, lover, sister or mother, on occasion, I will refer to the woman you care about as "she" or "her" – please don't take offence it just saves any confusion!

If you just want to dip in and out of the chapters, here is a quick overview of what lies ahead: the symptoms have been split into specific areas and within each chapter they are explained with advice on how to help manage them. Then follows a chapter with advice on lifestyle choices, diet and exercise – it's essential to look at all these areas being relevant not only for menopausal women but if addressed can help with many health issues, so giving a better quality of life long term and are relevant for both women and men. Hormone replacement therapy (HRT) is covered in Chapter 7 – the benefits and risks. Then the final chapter covers alternative remedies and therapies that can help with symptoms. Finally, there is a useful list of websites for signposting, websites which you can trust to have accurate, evidence-based information.

INTRODUCTION

In Menopause we are not ageing; we are ripening to perfection. (Indian Menopause Society)

So... she is going through the menopause. Gone is the calm, easy-going woman with the razor-sharp mind you once admired. In its place, an irritable, anxious and increasingly forgetful one.

Forget having an encyclopaedia living with you who could remember everyone's birthdays, what you had for supper three weeks last Friday, where you left your golf clubs and the year of that wonderful wine you had last week... to be replaced by a foggy brain and someone who bursts into tears at the drop of a hat. As for sex... well, let's move on quickly, shall we?

Any of this sound familiar?

Fear not! Everything you need to know about the female menopause is here in this handy guide. I've used easy-to-read layman's terms, minimum abbreviations and no mushy, gooey chat (you'll be relieved to hear). Just useful, relevant and practical information about what is potentially going on, how it will affect you, and how you can help. I'll cover everything from hot flush-es to vaginas, joint aches to libido... Settle! Having a nursing background, I'll dip into the medical stuff, but only that which is useful for you.

I'd like to take this opportunity to introduce Millie and Max who will accompany you throughout the book. Millie and Max are your average couple happily going through life. They have a good relationship with the usual ups and downs... that is until Millie started developing perimenopausal symptoms...

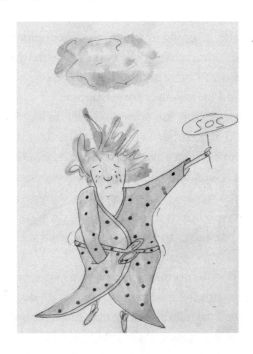

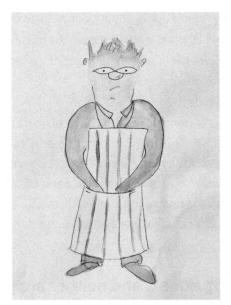

Let's start with a wonderful quote from a great friend of mine, now 60 years old and amongst the unfortunate generation of women who were largely denied the opportunity to have HRT because of the bonkers media hysteria and misinformation circa 2002. She's just a tad annoyed:

[The female menopause] is not talked about enough. If men's penises shrunk to the size of a date in their 50s, we'd have most of the Wellcome Foundation out there finding a cure for those poor "disenfranchised" men! Money would be diverted from saving pandas, the WWF would disintegrate, nobody would care about global warming, we would all be wading about the streets of London in wellies being told there's no money for tidal barriers... until there was A CURE!

She has a point – women have historically put up and shut up for far too long and it's only recently because of certain organisations (there are links to the ones I would recommend at the back of the book), and individuals raising awareness through various media channels that it has started to become more talked about.

She's not alone... and neither are you

Here's the first very important point to take on board: she is not alone or unusual.

Perimenopausal symptoms are very common, with approximately 80% of women suffering to some degree from a variety of symptoms. And there are reams of husbands and partners like you around the world trying to come to terms with this supposed new woman in your lives, when all you want is the old one back!

The main problem is that not enough people talk about it to normalise it, and there is definitely not enough consistent information given. This is improving but there still needs to be a lot more educating done right across the board.

1
SOME BASIC FACTS

The general perception of a menopausal woman needs to change – they should be valued for their wisdom and life experience and as such be acknowledged as an invaluable asset to society. (*Post Reproductive Health Journal* 2017)

So what is the menopause? How long does it last? Will she return to normal? Is the Pope a Catholic?… Of course she will!

Feel like you don't know anything? Please be assured you are not alone. There are thousands of men in exactly the same position as you, but alas, as a nation we tend to be all terribly British about it and we don't, as a rule, talk about it down the pub!

Here are a few definitions to start with:

- *Pre-menopause*: the reproductive phase, when the hormones are relatively intact.
- *Perimenopause*: that "glorious" transitional period from the reproductive phase to the non-reproductive phase, so potentially still fertile – careful! Oestrogen levels are declining and it can be a turbulent time for both of you. It's actually – and this is so important – the most

symptomatic phase, and for some can be flipping awful and for anyone in the vicinity!

- *Menopause/Post-menopause*: the non-reproductive phase, when periods have stopped (can only be classed as menopausal after 12 continual months of no bleeding). The symptoms should be dissipating and life starting to calm down... honest!
- *Prematurely menopausal*: a proportion of women can become menopausal before the age of 45, some in their 20s and 30s and for various reasons. These women should be on hormone replacement therapy (HRT) and should seek medical advice.

How, when and for how long?

Menopause can either be:
- *Spontaneous*, so developing naturally;
- *Surgically induced* following, for example, having a hysterectomy (symptoms tend to be more intense);
- *Iatrogenic* following treatment, as in chemotherapy or radiotherapy.

It usually starts to happen any time from the age of 45 to 55, the classic age quoted by clinicians being 51 years old.

How long can it last... how long is a piece of string? Anywhere between four and ten years is the average, but it is such an individual medical condition.

What's with all these symptoms? Does every woman get them?

Basically, all of the symptoms are due to declining levels of oestrogen. Every woman will go through this transitional phase but each woman will react differently.

Some sail through this transition; others find their symptoms so debilitating that it affects not only their general overall health but also their relationships and their work.

How can you help?

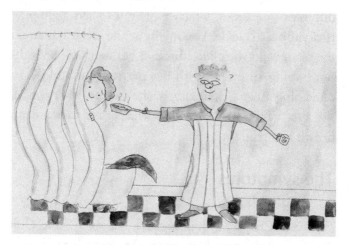

Firstly, a tip: never, and I mean *never*, say, "Oh it must be your hormones…", "Oh, it's definitely that time of month again…" or "Oh, go and take a chill pill…". These comments are like a red rag to a bull.

Do, however, send her off for long cool showers (soaks in the bath can, on occasion, exacerbate the hot flushes), be a model listener and learn to bite your tongue when required, even when she is resembling a Komodo dragon! This is absolutely no time for you to have any form of man flu! What do you mean, how long do you have to do this for?!

Over the following three chapters I'll go through symptoms that she *could* be experiencing and explain ways to help relieve those symptoms. Then, hopefully, quality of life will improve... for both of you.

The key word there is *could*. Most women experience several symptoms, but each woman is different, experiencing the symptoms in different ways and to different intensities, which is why it's such a flipping tricky topic to tackle! You might be the luckiest man on the planet and she glides through her menopause without batting an eyelid, with her pelvic floor and libido remaining intact. Alternatively, she's at the other end of the spectrum (sympathies), in which case, take a deep breath and read on...

The symptoms

I've split the main symptoms into three categories – *Physical* in Chapter 2, *Psychological* in Chapter 3 and *Genitourinary* in Chapter 4 (reproductive and urinary to you and me). There are also a few rare and long-term symptoms which you can find in Chapter 5.

OK, now brace yourself: there are over 30 symptoms that women can suffer from. Now you understand why she can resemble Cruella de Vil on occasion; there's a lot to cope with!

Always remember that certain symptoms could be related to other medical conditions, so if unsure, anyone should get checked out by their GP to confirm it is the menopause and not something else.

Something to take on board – symptoms evolve, some quicker than others and to differing degrees. Just when you think you've got a handle on everything, another one might rear its ugly head… but then again you might lose one! So it's a constant, ever-changing flow of events until reaching those post-menopausal years.

Symptoms & hormones

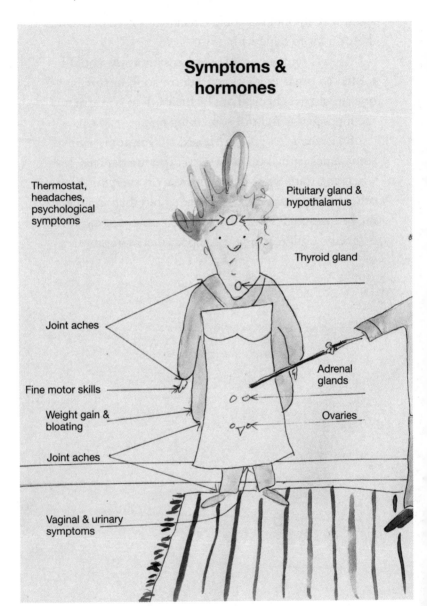

Pituitary gland: the 'master gland' which produces hormones that stimulate other glands to produce other hormones. It produces many hormones, two of them being luteinising hormone and follicle stimulating hormone which stimulate egg release and production of oestrogen by the ovaries.

Hypothalamus: controls many bodily functions including the release of hormones from the pituitary gland.

Thyroid gland: produces thyroid hormones which help to regulate the body's metabolic rate as well as heart and digestive function, muscle control, brain development, mood and bone maintenance.

Adrenal glands: attached to each kidney, they produce three hormones which help to regulate the body's salt and water levels, the body's metabolism and the production of testosterone (a percentage by the adrenal glands and a percentage by the ovaries).

Ovaries: produce and release eggs into the female reproductive system, they also produce the female hormones oestrogen and progesterone.

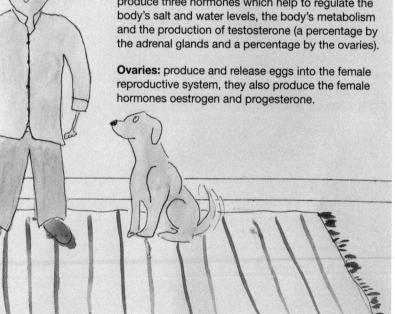

2
THE PHYSICAL SYMPTOMS

The human state includes far more than just the rational, analytical and intellectual behaviour based on physical objective facts but also includes the intuitive, the sensibilities and the spiritual. (*British Medical Journal* 2017 Margaret Turner-Warwick)

Everyone's heard of hot flushes, of course; she may even have started to experience these. But – brace yourself – there are many more physical symptoms that can accompany the onset of menopause. Read on to find out more about them, and what helps!

Hot flushes and night sweats

Hot flushes are the exact reverse of "feeling damn hot", I can assure you.

What happens?

The technical term is *vasomotor symptoms*. Hormones are all over the place as oestrogen levels start to drop, which causes the thermostat in the brain (that controls body temperature) to have a hissy fit now and again!

It affects 75% of women, with 25% getting really awful ones. That means she's either going to look like she's having "a wee glow" or like she's just come off a squash court – get the picture? I can assure you that they are inconvenient, embarrassing and disruptive, and they will affect her quality of life. They can be infuriatingly random and can also be brought on by certain foods, drinks or situations. It gets worse... they can be accompanied by headaches, palpitation and dizziness. Yes, we are still on the first symptom!

Triggers and causes

The most common triggers can be dietary, including caffeine, alcohol (with red wine being very common), spicy foods or even just having a hot drink.

Stressful situations can bring one on too, so what every woman needs from now on is peace, calm and tranquillity... I know that's not going to happen in the real world, but anything resembling peace and calm can help!

Other causes and/or triggers of flushes can be: certain cancer-related treatments, thyroid conditions, obesity, smoking and infection.

What can help?

- *Food and flush diary*: it sounds nerdy, but this is a good way to try and figure out which foods, drinks and situations are causing the worst symptoms and are potentially triggering the flushes. Then avoid or reduce the foods and drinks which trigger those flushes. Don't immediately go and put an order in for several cases of your favourite red – a little tact, please, boys!

- Encourage the wearing of *natural fibres*, i.e. cotton and bamboo fabrics, and get that bedroom well-ventilated. You might have to invest in some fleecy PJs for yourself!

- Drinking *plenty of water* and keeping hydrated is essential – replacing fluid after sweating a lot is a no brainer. The recommended daily intake is about two litres.

- With any symptom, lifestyle choices are going to get flagged up, meaning have a really good look at *diet and exercise* – that goes for both of you! Eating a healthy, nutritious diet and keeping well-hydrated helps all symptoms, as does doing a variety of exercise every week. No, don't go and sign her up for the local Ironman competition – little and often is fine. You can really help here: go for cycles, runs or walks together. Yes, you *do* have time, and you could earn major brownie points!

- *Cognitive behavioural therapy* (*CBT*) and *mindfulness*: there is a lot of research going on in these areas and both are definitely worth encouraging. No, it's not all airy-fairy mumbo-jumbo – positive thinking, learning simple CBT techniques and practicing mindfulness can really help to reduce the frequency and intensity of flushes. A good book to buy is *Managing Hot Flushes and Night Sweats* by Myra Hunter and Melanie Smith. (I should be on commission, the amount of women I've recommended this to!)

- *Herbal remedies* to consider include sage and black cohosh: always seek advice from a herbalist, though, as these can interact with other medications, and try to use ones which have the THR (Traditional Herbal Registration) logo (see Chapter 8 for more information).
- *Cooling Spray* by Promensil – sprayed on the skin, this helps to diffuse the heat.
- Look at products which can help wick moisture away from the body for example:
  - ◆ clothing – try bambooclothing.co.uk or cucucumberclothing.com
  - ◆ wool duvets – try southdownduvets.com

Medical treatment

Hormone replacement therapy – despite past scaremongering by the media, the benefits outweigh the risks and HRT helps enormously (see Chapter 7).

Any other medical options should be discussed in full with your GP and should be combined with lifestyle choices.

Palpitations

What happens?

Palpitations are heartbeats that can become noticeable. They are common, for most people are harmless and can often accompany hot flushes and night sweats. They can also be quite alarming and scary – if concerned always get checked out by your GP.

What can help?

As with the hot flushes and night sweats, relaxation and exercise are essential, plus learning those CBT techniques or trying some mindfulness.

Bleeding

Heavy bleeding – this can be debilitating, draining and life-changing.

What happens?

Some women develop very heavy periods accompanied, sometimes, by cramps and clots that can, on occasion, resemble a tsunami-like flow.

A large amount of women needlessly shut up and put up with these symptoms to detrimental effects, plus end up spending a fortune on sanitary products!

"Flooding", as it's sometimes known, can cause women to organise their holidays, social calendars and work diaries around their menstrual cycle which, quite frankly, can be so random and sporadic it's almost impossible to organise anything at all. She also won't buy or wear white jeans for quite a while!

At the other end of the spectrum, some women just gradually stop having periods without any heavy bleeding or complications at all. If she is in this group, she is very lucky... as are you!

What can help?

Medication

It's very important for any woman experiencing these symptoms to go and see her GP, to make sure it's hormonal fluctuations causing these symptoms and not some other reason. Once the cause is established and bloods have been taken to make sure you're not anaemic – which can be a side-effect of heavy menstruating – then your GP should discuss the various options to help with these symptoms.

Options available include:

- *non-hormonal medication,* which can help to reduce the flow of blood and can help with the cramps and clots: e.g. *mefenamic acid* or *tranexamic acid* can be prescribed;
- getting an intrauterine device fitted e.g. a *Mirena coil* (*releases progesterone*), which has the dual role of providing contraception as well as often having a miraculous effect on heavy bleeding;

- *oral progestogen* – taken cyclically, this helps regulate periods and can also help with flushes and sweats;
- *endometrial ablation*, a minor surgical procedure that can also have wonderful effects, like the coil.

Each of these options should be fully explained so every woman has the opportunity to make an informed and educated decision along with their GP as to the best route forward. Do encourage her to get her iron levels checked, as that can make her feel lethargic and worn out, but she definitely shouldn't self-medicate as too much iron isn't good for her either!

Important point: always get any unexplained bleeding checked out by your GP, especially if it's post-menopausal (after no periods for 12 months).

Lifestyle, diet and exercise

Having a healthy, nutritious, balanced diet with foods packed with iron is essential. Exercise definitely helps with cramps – often it's the last thing she will want to do, but try and encourage her to get active instead of curling up on the sofa with half of the M&S deli department!

You'll know she is on top of things when that first pair of white jeans reappears in her wardrobe.

Joint aches

What happens?

This is a very common symptom, mainly affecting wrists, neck, shoulders and hips. You often feel like your whole body resembles a creaking gate hanging off by its hinges! Getting out of the car, up from a chair or off a bike can feel like you're literally having to unfurl yourself into an upright position again.

Oestrogen plays an important role in helping to maintain joint and bone health, so when that starts fluctuating all over the place it makes sense that certain symptoms are going to appear.

Recognition of this symptom and associating it with menopause doesn't often happen; a lot of women think they are just getting old or that they have the start of arthritis (if in doubt, you can get a blood test to rule out rheumatoid arthritis).

What can help?

- *Exercise* – a lot of the time women will want to do the opposite: put their feet up to rest their aching joints, hug a hot water bottle because of their tummy cramps and seek out comfort food, whereas they should be doing the opposite on all fronts! A variety of exercise is good: *weight-bearing* (running), *non-weight-bearing* (cycling, swimming) and *resistance* (e.g. weights). Building *Pilates* or *yoga* into her week is incredibly useful. You too should join in on all these fronts, keeping that middle-aged spread at bay and staying supple.

- Developing a strong core really helps bone density and balance, which helps to reduce potential falls later in life – a no-brainer really. If she doesn't like conventional exercise, then try a different angle, such as dancing – those dancers on *Strictly* are some of the fittest people on the planet! Or do short sessions of HIIT (high intensity interval training – see Chapter 6).
- *Diet* – it's very important to have a diet rich in calcium, vitamin D and magnesium, so include foods such as oily fish, eggs, dairy products, green leafy vegetables, nuts and pulses in her diet.
- *Hydration* – lubricate those joints by drinking around two litres of water a day.
- *Relaxation* is good, and the odd massage is essential. You'll get major brownie points if you provide one of those… No, I don't mean you do it yourself; having a spa treatment can be heavenly!
- *Supplements* – if there is one supplement you should both take, it's vitamin D – 10 micrograms a day. With our climate here in the UK we just don't get enough sunshine, and then when we do go out in it we're probably plastered in Factor 30 sun cream!
- *Glucosamine* is a supplement to try; it occurs naturally and is one of the building blocks of cartilage. (It's also derived from shellfish, so be careful allergy wise.)

- *HRT* – this replaces lost oestrogen and has a good success rate of working on all symptoms. (See Chapter 7 for more information.)

Headaches

Headaches are another very common symptom of the perimenopause.

What happens?

Fluctuating hormones and changes in menstrual cycles (periods) can cause many women to experience "muzzy" heads, with some also experiencing migraines. And you thought she was just being a lightweight after a night out – not so! Having said that, I do believe alcohol tolerance reduces; but that little theory is not scientifically based, just my finding from speaking to hundreds of women! But back to headaches…

Once again, these symptoms are caused by fluctuating oestrogen. It's very common for women, regardless of their age, to experience cyclical headaches during their periods. Now you have an insight into what's been troubling your teenage daughter! So when going through the perimenopause with periods being all over the place, it can feel like you permanently have a headache.

The good news is that, if she gets her hot flushes, heavy bleeding and joint aches under control, more often than not the headaches will improve as she will now be exercising regularly, eating a wonderful healthy, nutritious diet, be hydrating madly and be engaging in an array of alternative therapies that you have been encouraging!

What can help?

- *Lifestyle choices* work here, with exercise really helping in some cases. It's a matter of figuring out what works for her as every woman will be different.
- *HRT* helps to regulate the hormones, so is very effective at helping with any menopausal symptom. However, some types of HRT can actually trigger a migraine (it's more likely with the oral/tablet form). If that is the case then it's a good idea to go back to your GP to discuss other options. Transdermal patches maintain a more stable delivery flow and are a recommended route for women experiencing migraines.
- *Non-hormonal medication* is available from your GP as well.

Weight gain and bloating

What happens?

Ah, the joys of the middle-aged spread! Contributed to with hormonal fluctuations and metabolic rates slowing down. It happens to many of us, you included, but practical lifestyle advice is at hand.

What can help?

- Keep a food diary

First and foremost, there are no benefits of faddy diets, taking diet pills or fasting continually. The best advice is to get that food diary on the go – as I said earlier, it sounds nerdy, but it can help both of you to focus on what you actually consume, how much, at what times of day; all of these things play a role in fat distribution. If she eats something that makes her feel bloated and you hear the odd trumping noise coming from the kitchen, then suggest she either reduces that particular food or takes it out of her diet altogether – it's not much fun for her if she's blowing up like a balloon!

- Make changes gradually

Slowly introduce different healthier foods into your diet, taking out or reducing the not-so-healthy ones, and subtly increasing exercise levels. Weight loss will happen in a sustainable way – it might be slower to happen, but will stand more chance of succeeding.

- Explore new diets

The Mediterranean and Asian countries have a lower incidence of cardiovascular disease, cancer rates, obesity and of menopausal symptoms being reported. I'm not saying you need to eat curry every night or munch on bean sprouts for the rest of your life but people in these countries do tend to have a more varied diet, cook from fresh, eat fewer convenience foods... get the idea?

- Have a rainbow plate

When thinking about food, think "rainbow". I'm serious – the more colourful, the better. Instead of counting calories, count the nutrients! (See Chapter 6 for more advice on a healthy diet.)

- Slow down and digest

When eating, you should both eat little and often, plus try to slow down the pace of eating – this seriously helps! Also, add foods such as ginger that aid digestion into recipes. Don't forget to hydrate, too – it always helps.

- Some things you can't change

However, it's not all about what you eat – as you get older your metabolic rate can slow down and the way your body distributes fat can change. The classic pear-shaped woman can then start to resemble more of a Granny Smith apple, with a widening of the midriff. Do have a quick glance down at yourself, though, as it can happen to men too. The difference for women is that the fluctuating hormones are playing their role in all of this, too, and that part is frustratingly out of their control!

Note: If someone is desperate to kick-start a change in their diet by fasting and you can't change their mind, suggest the best natural way to achieve a fasting period is to eat your last meal early, so say 6 pm, then don't have anything to eat until breakfast at 7 am the next morning... a natural 12-hour fast whilst maintaining regular nutritious eating during the day!

Insomnia and fatigue

Not surprisingly, these are two of the most common symptoms and trying to get a good night's sleep can become all-consuming, and it's not helped by you snoring or grinding your teeth next to her!

What happens?

If she's got even half of the previous symptoms she's probably not sleeping properly. She might be waking up with night sweats, struggling to keep hydration levels up, maybe she's anaemic – you get the picture.

What can help?

Addressing and getting on top of all the other symptoms will help, as will the following:

- exercise
- hydration
- having earlier meal times
- establishing a calming bedtime routine, with no techie stimulation (laptops, phones, TVs) in the room. I'm not going to suggest that whale music be piped into your bedroom every night, but... you never know, it might work!

The more relaxed, well-nourished and exercised she is, the better her body will cope with the symptoms.

Every little thing that she tries can help, and an exercised, rested and relaxed woman will sleep better. End result – she feels less irritable and crabby, and everyone's happy!

Fine motor skills

Some women find that they become more clumsy, dropping things on occasion. From her point of view it's another annoying symptom to add to the list, and it's not helped by disparaging looks and rolling eyes from other parties – especially those hormonal teenage children... It's one of the short-term symptoms, though, so hopefully she won't get round to dropping that priceless Ming vase!

With any symptom, if she's in any doubt that it could be related to another medical condition, she needs to see her GP rather than self-diagnosing or self-medicating.

3
THE PSYCHOLOGICAL SYMPTOMS

If you're absent during my struggle, don't expect to be present during my success. (Will Smith)

Brain ache

Common phrases associated with the psychological symptoms are "Brain fog" and "Red Mist", which both aptly describe how sometimes your brain can feel during the perimenopause; like it's wading through treacle!

When I get onto these symptoms during a menopause workshop, I can see the sheer relief pass over women's faces when they realise that they are not the only ones suffering from these symptoms and that – hurrah – they are not going completely bonkers after all!

Psychological symptoms have to be some of the most debilitating, frustrating and misunderstood symptoms of the menopause, being amongst some of the least talked about, as with most mental health issues.

Bizarre, isn't it? As a society we feel comfortable talking about physical symptoms, whereas with anything remotely psychological we all tend to keep our heads down, which makes everything ten times as hard to cope with. Don't underestimate the effect hormone fluctuations might be having.

The most common symptoms which can be experienced are low mood swings (very different from full-blown depression), anger and irritability, forgetfulness, poor concentration and anxiety – which can progress with some women to develop into panic attacks.

What happens?

As with all of the symptoms associated with the menopause, oestrogen deficiency (so fluctuating hormones) plays a huge role in causing these symptoms. I say "a huge role", as other contributing factors also play their parts. External pressures contribute enormously and shouldn't be discounted. For example, we are often referred to as "the sandwich generation" within a family, squidged in between those equally hormonal teenage children (who come with their own set of challenges, the little darlings!) and our ageing parents, who can become increasingly challenging too, but in different ways.

So it's no wonder that, with all this to cope with, and the added stress of those flipping, fluctuating hormones getting thrown into the mix that women often feel a tad under pressure. They may, as a result, get angry and irritable, display irrational, out-of-character behaviour and have heightened emotional sensitivity. This is ALL completely normal and understandable. DO I MAKE MYSELF CLEAR?!

Millie has a few of the psychological symptoms going on… this diagram shows the most commonly experienced psychological symptoms, and options which can help treat or lessen those symptoms.

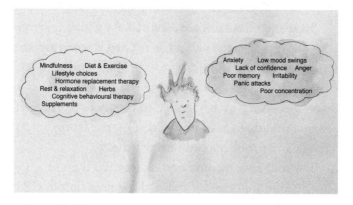

What helps?

OK, now we've established she's not going loop-the-loop, you can breathe a sigh of relief. However, please do not adopt a patronising attitude because you're pleased at having worked out the cause… No, she requires understanding, copious amounts of TLC and, most importantly, support to address those lifestyle choices. I know I'm banging on about these again, but I can't emphasise enough how making tweaks to anyone's diet and exercise can make the most significant difference to a multitude of health issues. It's never too late to start, and never too early either; yes, you too!

What you eat can make a significant difference to how you feel – incorporating more energising foods, reducing the carbs, eating only the healthy fats and keeping hydrated are all so important. Exercise plays a huge role when coping with any psychological symptom – try to incorporate a variety of exercise into each week alongside either Pilates or yoga sessions.

Rest and relaxation are essential. As with any symptom, the less stressed and more relaxed women are, the less intense their symptoms will be, having the knock-on effect of you being less stressed too! Just being given the luxury of being able to think about yourself for one minute instead of the rest of the family's busy agenda and problems can seriously help.

I would also recommend alternative therapies, including mindfulness and CBT. Learning simple CBT coping mechanisms can help enormously to develop a more positive way of thinking. It's not a quick fix but definitely something to consider, learning techniques which are then transferable to help cope with other symptoms. See Chapter 8 for more information on alternative therapies.

Medication

There's a range of medication, both conventional and alternative, to look into:

- *HRT* doesn't just help the physical symptoms; it can really help the psychological ones as well.

Often when HRT has helped to sort the draining physical ones out, women then have more energy to think clearly and tackle the ones they probably didn't even realise they were suffering from.

- *Anti-depressants* (selective scrotonin reuptake inhibitors (SSRIs)): the NICE guidelines* say that these should not be used as a first line of treatment. They definitely have their place in the medical and menopause world, but in the past have sometimes been handed out like sweeties by GPs the moment an emotional, flushing woman enters their surgery. GPs have such a tricky job keeping abreast of so many different specialties and, what with the ridiculously short time slots allotted to appointments, you can't really blame them in some respects, but unfortunately there has been a touch of over-prescribing in this area.

- *Alternatives, such as herbs*: tread with caution and always consult a trained herbalist. Just because something is a herb doesn't mean it's not going to have side effects − for example, one of the most commonly used herbs for low mood is St John's Wort, but this can interact with various conventional medicines and is very potent.

- *Supplements*: try to make sure she doesn't dash off into that well-known supplement retail outlet to buy a variety of herbs and supplements and start taking a random combination just because her neighbour three doors down has found one or two that work. She won't be able to identify which one is working, and mixing up a cocktail of herbs and supplements without experienced advice can have unwanted side effects. And she's got enough to cope with!

- *Foods rich in B12 and Omega 3*: because low levels of vitamin B12 and Omega 3 can increase feelings of low mood. But instead of immediately going to buy supplements, a healthier option is to make sure diets incorporate foods which are rich in these nutrients – oily fish, whole grains and flax seeds all help, as well as nutritional yeast with added B12. You should be able to get enough through having a healthy diet.

On a lighter note, as with other relatively short-term symptoms, once her hormones start to behave themselves, the psychological symptoms should start to calm down and the person you know and love will return back to normal... or she'll become a newer, happier version of herself!

4
THE GENITOURINARY SYMPTOMS (REPRODUCTIVE AND URINARY)

Women's healthcare must focus on preventing ill health,
rather than fire-fighting disease. (NHS 2011)

Let's talk vaginas

I know, it's a seriously unappealing term, and not terribly sexy, but it basically means "reproductive and urinary" to us lay folk.

As with the psychological symptoms, these symptoms really aren't talked about enough. Let's face it, it's not the first topic to come up when out for a beer with your pals! A large proportion of the female population is not even comfortable saying the word "vagina", so they tend to adopt pet names for their nether regions – Fi-Fi, muff, foo-foo, and the like. Personally, I will never be able to look at an orchid in the same way again after a friend told me her 70-year-old mother said that orchids always remind her of vaginas!

However, I would like to tell every woman I meet to LOVE YOUR VAGINA! A leaflet should be put through every woman's letterbox stating this and then explaining why. I often say to women that they should give as much attention to their vaginas as their faces – seriously! We spend so much money on facial products, pampering spa treatments, and so on, all because we can see our faces and they are on public view. Whereas vaginas require just as much attention but are, for obvious reasons, not on show (I admit that would be a step too far!). So they just don't receive the same levels of care and attention. Sadly, I come across an incredible amount of women who have resigned themselves – and their partners – to a predominantly asexual life, and who put up with symptoms that can often be remedied easily.

What happens?

By now you'll be familiar with the term, Oestrogen Deficiency – as well as all of the other physical and psychological symptoms, it can also cause and contribute to:

- *Vaginal atrophy* – thinning and wasting away of tissues in that area. The ideal is plump with wrinkles (agree, slightly different from what she wants for her facial tissue!).
- *Vaginal irritation, dryness and soreness* – all contribute to painful, uncomfortable intercourse.

- *Vaginal infections* – changes in the acidity levels makes some women more prone to infections.
- *Urinary problems* such as frequency, urgency and leakage.
- *Reduced sex drive and loss of libido* – this is very common. There could, of course, be other contributing factors – I mean HOW long have you two known each other? Would you say you have remained sexually appealing?! Just putting that out there – it's not all about her, you know, this is a two-way thing!

Symptoms will require long-term treatment, so it makes sense to get them sorted. It's said that up to 40% of women are affected. Personally, from speaking to so many women over the years I think that percentage is higher; it just goes unreported.

What can help?

First, you have to tactfully get her to admit she has a problem. I'll leave that one up to you because you know her best, but it can be a tricky road, so tread carefully. Here are some useful tips:

- Check out said vagina (I mean her, not you)

If you can get her to check her vagina out, that would be handy. I come across a remarkable amount of women who never have a gander down there, don't know what is normal for them and just want to ignore the whole issue, the result being no sex, extreme discomfort and a life with Tena pads looming on the horizon!

- Vaginal moisturisers and lubricants

These are brilliant inventions. A simple moisturiser can immediately soothe dryness, help to relieve irritation and help with lubrication during intercourse. There is a vast array on the market, it's just a matter of finding one which suits you. One I would recommend is a company called Sylk. They not only have delightful staff to deal with, but their product is also fabulous. Classed as a moisturising lubricant, it is prescribable on the NHS or you can just go online and order it direct. It's non-hormonal, paraben-free and guess what – it works!

- Vaginal oestrogen

If vaginal moisturisers have been tried and her symptoms persist, then it can be a good idea to go and see your GP to discuss the option of being prescribed vaginal oestrogen which comes in a variety of forms including pessaries, creams, gels or an oestrogen ring which is inserted into the vagina for three months at a time and slowly releases oestrogen. Each different type of application gives excellent results.

The beauty of vaginal oestrogen is that it goes directly to where it is needed, contains only a tiny amount of oestrogen and has very low systemic absorption – handy if anyone's worried about taking hormones (do look at Chapter 7, though). And it seriously works. Not only does it help with vaginal symptoms but think how close the vagina and urethra are... yes... it helps with urinary leakage, frequency and urgency, too.

- Pelvic floor exercises

These really help with urinary symptoms; and after all, women should not have to resign themselves to years of using Tena pads. Plus, if she gets that pelvic floor into shape, she (and you) should experience better orgasms. Squeezy* is a brilliant app to download. It's developed by physiotherapists specialising in women's health and explains everything you need to know about pelvic floors, plus it gives great exercise routines.

And, for those of you chaps who don't realise – you, too, have a pelvic floor that needs exercised. Yes, I'm deadly serious! Off you go – get exercising!

- Exercise

Not again, I hear you cry! It really helps, though. Pilates and yoga are essential as you can't help but do pelvic floor exercises during the course of a class.

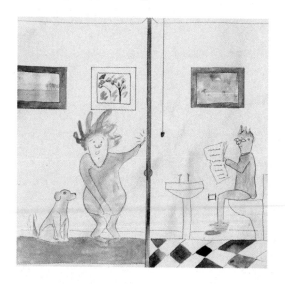

5
RARE AND POSSIBLE LONG-TERM SYMPTOMS

If you are willing to do only what's easy, life will be hard.
But if you're willing to do what is hard, life will be easy.
(T. H. Eker)

We're nearly at the end of the symptoms – we just have a few more to look at, these are the rare and possible long-term symptoms.

Rare symptoms

There are a few classic rare symptoms and then some absolutely bizarre ones which, alas, have no research behind them so I can't really put them down here, but they do crop up in conversation now and again. (Ever heard of Electric Leg?!) Here are some of the more well-documented rare symptoms:

- *Burning Mouth Syndrome*: this can feel like you've scalded your mouth, with some women experiencing multiple mouth ulcers. Not surprisingly, taste buds can be affected.

- *Dental sensitivity*: don't worry, her teeth aren't going to drop out, but she might experience more sensitivity in her gums and teeth.
- *Thinning hair*: this is age-related as well as hormone-related – have a look at the top of your head some time! Unfortunately it can affect a large proportion of the female population.
- *Formication* (not fornication!): this can feel like insects are crawling on your skin – it's very itchy.

Treatment

As with all symptoms, these are down to oestrogen deficiency. The best way to help them is through lifestyle choices – a healthy, nutritious diet and plenty of exercise (see Chapter 6). All can be helped by taking HRT (see Chapter 7).

Possible long-term symptoms

As with any medical condition, not every woman will develop these symptoms. I'm sure the media would love to stir up the nation as it did with HRT and make us think we're all going to start developing crumbling bones and have several fractures and heart attacks each by the time we reach 70. Thankfully, it would be fairly obvious if every second person you came across was on crutches or collapsing in the street. Luckily that's not going to happen, so let's move on from the media's scaremongering to look at the long-term symptoms which some *may* experience.

Osteoporosis: low bone density

It's known as the silent disease and is often only diagnosed when someone has a fall resulting in a fracture. We all lose bone density, as part of getting older, but women can tend to lose density more rapidly with the decline of oestrogen, as oestrogen helps to conserve bone and absorb calcium. We definitely drew the short straw in life on this one! If worried about levels of bone density, anyone can check online using a programme called FRAX*. Or if there is a family history of say, for example, hip or wrist fractures, then it might be an idea to be referred by your GP for a Dexa scan* which measures bone mineral density levels.

Important point: women are more at risk of developing osteoporosis if menopause is premature – so before the age of 45 years.

Cardiovascular symptoms

Oestrogen has a protective effect on the cardiovascular system so, with declining levels, just be aware of this. With osteoporosis and cardiovascular symptoms, as with any health conditions, prevention is better than fire-fighting so, yes, it's back to lifestyle choices, diet and exercise!

What can help?

- A variety of *regular exercise* helps to strengthen bones and helps to keep that heart healthy.

- *Pilates and yoga* not only help to strengthen bones but help with balance, so reducing the risk of falling.
- Eating a *healthy, nutritious diet* which has plenty of calcium and vitamin D is good for your bones, and also include magnesium for your heart.
- If there's one supplement we should all be taking it's *vitamin D*, 10 micrograms per day. Yes, that includes you too!
- *Give up smoking* and *be aware of alcohol intake*. Fear not, I am not going to tell anyone to give up alcohol completely and become teetotal, most of us need a wee tipple now and then. If you are in any doubt about your levels, though, go on the Drink Aware website* and fill in the questionnaire – you will soon find out!

Genitourinary symptoms are also classed as a long-term symptom; see Chapter 4 for information about these.

6
LIFESTYLE, DIET AND EXERCISE

The aim of medicine is to prevent disease and prolong life, the ideal of medicine is to eliminate the need for a physician. (William James Mayo 1861–1939)

This chapter is devoted entirely to the natural ways to cope with whatever symptoms might be rearing their ugly heads – the ones she realises she has and the others that you (gently) might have to point out she's suffering from, both physical and psychological. Ultimately, though, it's a good time to choose to live a better, healthier life.

All those positive lifestyle choices I've been banging on about through the last five chapters can make such a difference to overall health, not just menopausal symptoms. So you, too, will benefit from reading these pearls of wisdom, a lot of which are just good old common sense.

It's easier together

As with anything to do with lifestyle choices, the hardest things are, first, admitting that your lifestyle choices need a bit of tweaking and, second, to motivate yourself to make those changes and put into practice what you know you should be doing. If you do this together, it will be a lot easier (just saying… do stop groaning!).

Alcohol

Let's start with alcohol. You both might be teetotal, of course (if that's the case, move quickly on to the next point), but steeped as we are in the British pub culture, more often than not I come across women who like the odd tipple, and when the going gets tough, for example:

- they've had a stressful day at work forgetting things, dropping things, flushing constantly throughout an important board meeting;
- they got caught out with not enough sanitary products whilst in said meeting;
- they missed their lunch-break due to having to dash to Boots for sanitary products;
- they have to cope with demanding teenagers when they get home…
- when they finally reach home, the first thing they do is reach for that bottle of wine chilling in the fridge that they popped in there the night before. What on earth is wrong with that, you might say, as you join them and share that bottle before supper, and then as you reach for the second bottle of red warming by the fire…?

Everything in moderation ... (ah I know so dull, but needs must!)

Alcohol in moderation is absolutely fine, but it can exacerbate symptoms, for example red wine is well known for triggering hot flushes.

Having too much alcohol is also linked with certain cancers and obesity. It does not help with mental health issues and can contribute to making those perimenopausal symptoms much worse – more intense and frequent hot flushes, weight gain, bloating, headaches and insomnia. It's not good for bone density either.

So, little and often is OK if it's within the guidelines but, seriously, cut out any binge drinking!

What are the guidelines?

Government guidelines say that we should not be having more than 14 units of alcohol a week and it's much better for your body to spread those 14 units throughout the week and not have them in a oner!

What does the government know, I hear you say? In my workshops, I commonly hear things like, "My granny used to drink at least four gin-and-tonics every night, lived 'til she was 93 years old and was as fit as a flea." There's always the exception to the rule but, for the majority of us, excessive alcohol does contribute to health issues and, as ever, prevention is better than fire-fighting. We can't see what is going on on a daily basis with our arteries, bones and livers – we only find out if something is amiss when we start to get symptoms. It's much better, I'm sure you'd agree, to try and get lifestyle choices sorted out, and to make sure a better quality of life is achieved... no?!

Top alcohol tips

- Always have a glass of water with a drink; hydrate as you go!
- Reduce the size of wine glass you both use – e.g. go from a 175 ml glass to a 125 ml glass of wine.
- If either of you drinks pints of beer or cider, have the odd half... wean yourselves off gently, so it's sustainable.
- Be realistic, and if you do drink regularly, then try and have the odd alcohol-free night every week as well. You'll more than likely get a better sleep!

Smoking

If either of you smoke, try to stop, or reduce. Everyone knows it is a health risk, associated with cardiovascular problems and cancers. It also inhibits absorption of medication and nutrients and can exacerbate many of her symptoms – no-brainer to stop really...

Diet

A lot of women complain they are still eating the same foods and doing the same levels of exercise they have always done, yet they seem to be putting on weight. Well, that's partly because those hormones are having a field day in there, creating havoc not only with mood swings and hot flushes, but with weight distribution, water retention… you name it, they are up to no good!

It's time to nudge the diet and exercise in opposite directions. Have a really good look at what you both eat, and, try to identify which foods are triggering certain symptoms (keeping a food diary is really useful, even for just a few days). There isn't a "menopausal diet" but here are some handy tips…

Eat a healthy, nutritious, balanced diet including at least *five portions of fruit and veg* per day.
Focus on *counting nutrients* rather than calories.
Don't skip meals – it makes it harder to achieve your nutritional requirements or to maintain a healthy weight. And *avoid faddy diets*; anything she does has to be sustainable and for the long term.
Little and often is ideal – keep that metabolic rate ticking over.
Have *healthy snacks* to hand such as almonds, dried apricots, apples, carrot sticks and peppers. Before you both screw your faces up, just try them! They're packed with nutrients and are heaps better for you than a chocolate bar.
Really *notice* what you are putting into your body; the more *variety*, the better.
Eat *fresh rather than processed*. Aim for calories which are packed with nutrients rather than empty ones which just give you a quick sugar rush and nothing else.

Nuts, seeds (e.g. flaxseed) and *green vegetables* (e.g. spinach, kale, green beans) are essential.

Vary your fruit and veg! Don't stick to the same one or two varieties — every week, try to introduce something new you haven't tried before. Think a rainbow of food; the more colourful, the better.

Try to *avoid convenience foods* and incorporate more unrefined foods, such as wholegrains (brown bread, rice, bran cereal), fruits and vegetables.

Reduce alcohol and caffeine. If caffeine is triggering certain symptoms, try cutting down, or drink alternatives such as herbal teas or decaf coffee.

Always *hydrate* throughout the day – aim for two litres of water a day on top of your coffee and tea.

Try to massively *reduce sugar and refined carbohydrate intake.* But don't be completely grim, give yourself a tiny treat every day – e.g. a bite-sized piece of dark chocolate (70–75% cocoa) instead of a morning pastry or fruit scone in the afternoon. I've been there, done that and know the pitfalls!

Healthy fats are essential, as are complex carbs such as wholegrain foods, oatmeal, beans and peas. You need all these for energy.

Eat *unsaturated fats* (oils, nuts, oily fish), *not saturated* (butter, cream, lard, fatty cuts of meat) and *avoid trans fats* at all costs – they have no nutritional value and are harmful to health.

Have a look at your cooking methods. *Steaming* is better than frying, as it helps to retain vitamins and minerals. Try *poaching* instead of frying eggs, *grill* things rather than frying, and *stir-fry* rather than always using sauces.

Try to incorporate foods into her diet that are rich in *phytoestrogens* (plant substances that have effects similar to oestrogen) – they include cereals, seeds, pulses, beans and soya.

To help maintain *healthy bones* in particular, eat foods rich in *calcium* and *vitamin D*:

- oily fish (salmon and sardines)
- eggs
- dairy products such as milk (whole or semi-skimmed is best!) and yogurts – natural ones are the best without additives and sugar, and you can add fresh fruit if you need a flavour

To help maintain a *healthy heart*, follow these tips:

- Cut down on saturated fats, replacing with unsaturated fats, e.g. swap butter for olive oil and have natural yogurt, or non-dairy alternative, instead of cream.
- Try to incorporate oily fish into your diet at least twice a week – sardines, salmon and mackerel are all good sources.

• cheese • green leafy vegetables e.g. kale, broccoli, spinach • nuts, seeds, dried fruit are all good sources • flax seeds and tofu are essential additions if vegan.	• Make sure you are getting lots of fibre – think wholegrain, pulses such as lentils and beans, plenty of fruit and vegetables. • Calm down on the salt intake – ideal is less than 6g per day. • If you eat meat, try to stick to lean cuts.

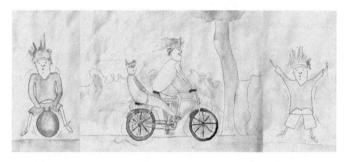

Exercise

Engaging in some form of exercise will help any symptom. The ideal being to do a variety of exercise throughout the week: aerobic, weight-bearing and resistance, including essential core work.

Cycling, swimming, running, dancing, tennis and netball are all great. Try and incorporate a Pilates or a yoga class once a week – and why not you as well? You have a core, too, and a pelvic floor that needs toning (download the brilliant Squeezy* app for essential tips and exercises).

Join the HIIT parade

If she doesn't like conventional exercise, avoids gyms and hates Lycra, then suggest just 10 minutes of HIIT (high intensity interval training to you and me). If done properly it is comparable to 30 minutes of aerobic exercise, plus you can roll out of bed and do it in the comfort and privacy of your own home!

HIIT is "short bursts of intense exercise, followed by timed, less intense periods of recovery". That doesn't mean you run on the spot flat out for 10 minutes, which could result in collapsing in a heap and never trying again. Try splitting it up into 1 minute of exercise followed by 30 seconds of recovery sections. Plus in the 30-second recovery time fit in doing a pelvic floor squeeze (women like a bit of multitasking!).

Have fun – go for a bounce

And make it fun, so it's sustainable. To some people, fun means burpees and squats, but to me fun means skipping (which tests the pelvic floor too), or even bouncing on a space-hopper (yes, you can get adult ones that give you an intense thigh workout – and you could have a morning race with her!). Just use your imagination and choose a combination that is going to inspire you both to exercise at least three times a week … how about starting that Salsa class?!

Make positivity the goal

Set sustainable, realistic goals and not only will weight levels reduce (if needed), it will also help any symptom to reduce in intensity and frequency, helps anyone feel more positive and able to cope.

That, in turn, helps with those psychological symptoms, which means she can make more measured decisions on how to cope with the trickier symptoms if medication is needed.

Why all of this is important

The bottom line is that obesity is an increasing global problem and is a recognised factor in many serious diseases, including breast cancer and endometrial cancer. It is never too late to start exercising and eating healthily. It can be hard to get motivated, but if you give her (and yourself) heaps of encouragement, and try to be organised, it'll be easier to stick to your exercise and eating plans.

7
HORMONE REPLACEMENT THERAPY (HRT)

There should be a holistic and individualised approach in assessing menopausal women with particular reference to lifestyle advice, diet modification as well as discussing the role of HRT.
(*Post Reproductive Health Journal* December 2016)

Will she or won't she? Does she really need it? What are the risks? Should I believe the media? Does it work?

My personal views about HRT, which are mirrored by many women I have met and worked with who have taken it, is that its effects can be almost miraculous. But everyone is obviously unique so for something as complex as the topic of HRT, each woman should have the opportunity to be treated holistically and individually, resulting in being able to make an educated decision with the help of their HCP.

There are many factors to take into consideration, such as individual physiology, medical history and all the pros and cons of taking HRT. It's all about having access to comprehensive, evidence-based information, so you can then make that educated decision.

Looking at it from a different angle... imagine it in terms of a flat tyre on a car... it causes the car to drive poorly, maybe even dangerously. That tyre needs air so you replace the air. The car's back on track, safe and working as it should be.

Similarly, a woman's body *can* suffer from greatly reduced levels of oestrogen. It can cause horrible, often life-altering symptoms, so it surely makes sense to replace that oestrogen (individual medical circumstances obviously need to be taken into consideration).

The important information

There is so much information I could give you, but I've tried to stick to the crucial bits. I've also included some respected, evidence-based websites with more detailed information – the links are at the end of the book – as I know how concerned some women remain about the safety of HRT and all those pros and cons.

A few key points

Diagnosis should be from *symptoms alone*, not by having an FSH (follicle stimulating hormone) test, *unless* prematurely menopausal, i.e. 45 years and under. Oh, and *saliva tests are a waste of money* – have a shopping spree instead!	All women should be treated *holistically* and *individually*, and it should be explained about the advantages and necessities of addressing lifestyle choices including diet, exercise, alcohol intake and caffeine levels.

If symptoms are not being controlled by adjustments to lifestyle choices alone, and your lives are being affected, that is a sign that she might want to consider *HRT* or some other form of medication.	The *pros and cons*, benefits and risks of taking HRT should be discussed, as should the options of the different *delivery routes* available.
HRT consists of *oestrogen* and *progesterone* – the progesterone is there to protect the endometrial lining of the uterus. If she's had a hysterectomy she does not need the progesterone part.	The *non-hormonal medical alternatives* and the other alternatives available, e.g. herbal remedies, should all be discussed as well (see Chapter 9).

Will your primary-care clinician have time to discuss all of this? Probably not – it usually takes at least an hour, hence the need for this book!

What does HRT do for her?

- HRT can help with a wide range of menopausal symptoms and is definitely the most effective treatment available.
- HRT has potential cardio-protective effects if taken within 10 years of starting perimenopausal

symptoms (this is known as the "window of opportunity").

- HRT helps to prevent and treat other potential long-term symptoms of oestrogen deficiency such as osteoporosis. It contributes to the maintenance of bone density, so helping to reduce the risk of osteoporotic fractures.
- Additional benefits may include helping to reduce the occurrence of colorectal cancer, Type 2 diabetes and Alzheimer's. More research is needed within these areas, but the current picture is positive.

What about the risks?

- The cardiovascular risk for the average woman should not be increased when starting HRT under the age of 60 and for some women under expert medical care they can remain on low doses of HRT indefinitely.
- In relation to the breast cancer risk, the latest research at time of writing states that HRT acts as a *promotor* rather than an *initiator*, meaning that the HRT could accelerate the progression of breast cancer cells already present. You are much more likely to increase the risk of getting cancer if you drink excessive amounts of alcohol or if you are obese. That's why I've been banging on about the importance of lifestyle choices, diet and exercise.
- The benefits outweigh the risks.

When should you take it and for how long?

- If any woman is prematurely menopausal (before the age of 45), they need to be on HRT until at least the classic age of 51 years – end of story.
- If you're prescribed HRT, it should be reviewed after three months, and then six months, then annually – from experience, when it goes onto annual review she will probably have to keep up to date with that herself. The same seems to happen in some practices with Mirena coil replacement – I've met women with them in still unreplaced after 10 years. Please note – they are licensed for just 5 years' use for contraception purposes and 4 years for providing HRT.
- There is a misconception that you should start taking HRT only once your periods have stopped. That's not the case – HRT can be taken in the perimenopausal stage if symptoms require it.
- Women can be prescribed HRT indefinitely as long as other contributory factors are taken into account and they are reviewed annually (see NICE guidelines*).

Contraception...

When, after 12 continual months of no periods, she is finally classed as being menopausal, there is still a slim chance of her becoming pregnant! I know; how bonkers does that seem? Don't take risks, guys, and make sure contraception is in place for up to two more years if 51 years and under and for one more year if over the age of 51 years… well, it's up to you but if you don't want to hear the pitter-patter of tiny feet in your retirement then it's a no-brainer!

How is HRT administered?

Oral

Tablets are the most common way to get HRT. They're cost-effective and they treat many symptoms.

Transdermal (through the skin)

This comes as a patch or in a gel. It's a better delivery system all round. It's much better for women who suffer from migraines/headaches. But they're more expensive, so if your GP isn't offering this type, just ask for it!

Implant

This can be injected beneath the skin which provides a slow release of oestrogen over several months – less common route.

Vaginal

Systemic HRT can be prescribed (HRT for her whole body rather than localised HRT) and, in addition, the vaginal HRT if required. Some women have horrendous symptoms in this area that the systemic HRT just doesn't hit home with. It is very common to have vaginal oestrogen prescribed as well and it is safe to do so.

Important note: there are many different preparations of HRT and one type does not suit everyone. If one has been tried and it doesn't suit, then it is very likely that it will be possible to find another type that will suit, so persevere. And remember, a prescription is only as good as the prescriber's knowledge – so make sure she sees someone who knows what they are talking about!

Why might she not take HRT?

Even after reading all the above, trawling through numerous websites and chatting to her GP, she might not fancy HRT, and that is absolutely her decision.

Or she might have tried HRT by now and she's not tolerated it – occasionally some women have side effects.

HRT might not be medically advised, however, for example if there is a previous history of breast cancer, or cardiovascular problems such as a stroke. All past medical history should be taken into account.

Are there any alternatives?

There are several *medications* available which GPs can prescribe. Again, it's down to medical history and personal preference.

These are *non-hormonal medical alternatives*, but they tend to only treat a couple of symptoms, whereas HRT treats a whole umbrella of symptoms.

For reduced levels of libido, *testosterone* is presently not licensed for use in the UK but can be prescribed by menopause specialists in certain circumstances. Regular systemic HRT helps enormously in this area, though, so give it a bit of time.

A word of warning...

There are hormonal treatments called *bio-identical hormones*, these are "compounded" which means they are basically made to order and often use hormones which are not approved for use in women. These are not regulated or subject to any quality control, and they cost a lot. Far better to organise a weekend away instead, and only use regulated medication.

Progesterone cream is another one which can be bought over the internet – again, don't bother as it's not absorbed well, you can't tell how much progesterone you are getting and it does not provide the necessary protection for the endometrial lining if taking oestrogen.

Essentially, please don't buy hormonal medication, or any medication for that matter, off the internet, always see your GP or a recognised menopause specialist. The British Menopause Society have recently added a list of menopause specialists which you can be directed to using your postcode.

So there you have it – a whistle-stop tour of HRT! If you would like to read up on it in depth, check out the links at the end of the book.

8
ALTERNATIVE REMEDIES AND THERAPIES

All things are poison for there is nothing without poison-
ous qualities. It is the dose which makes a thing a poison!
(Paracelsus 1577)

What if she doesn't fancy hormones or other forms of medication? Don't despair – there are alternatives.

I felt that the pages of this chapter should be im-pregnated with those wonderful smells you inhale on entering a spa, which immediately send anyone into re-laxation mode. My first top tip is to go and buy some essential oils or one of those smelly candles – you'll be amazed at the results! Apparently geranium oil is a good one for the menopause.

Here are a few points to remember when taking alternative remedies, whether they are individual herbs, simple supplements or complex supplements:

- They can be effective but are not entirely risk-free.
- There are concerns as to methods of produc-tion and quality control.

- The choice is completely and utterly confusing and bamboozling, so always seek advice from a qualified, experienced therapist. Do NOT randomly pick products off a shelf just because your friend said it worked!
- There is a lack of evidence from randomised trials that alternative and complementary therapies improve menopausal symptoms or have the same benefits as HRT. In addition, more often than not these companies can't afford to have the clinical trials either.
- Herbal remedies are treated as food supplements so are not subjected to the same strict regulations as conventional drugs.
- Many people don't realise that there is concern over the interaction with conventional medicines. Herbs can be very strong and many interact with prescribed drugs.
- There is an EU directive on traditional herbal products which *doesn't* cover products bought outside Europe, so don't go and buy any medication or supplement off the internet.
- Some herbs are not recommended for women who have had breast cancer as they have oestrogenic properties.

OK, now you know that alternative remedies should be treated with caution – so let's have a look at how to safely use herbal remedies.

Herbal remedies

- These definitely have their place in the treatment of menopausal symptoms, but use them wisely and be aware of the previous points.
- Read the back of the packet and check the contents; lots of companies put in fillers/packers.
- If she does go down the herbal route, she should try to speak to a phytotherapist/herbalist who not only will give advice on which herbs to recommend but will know which pharmaceutical medications interact with the herbal remedies. If one isn't available, it's best to try one herb at a time rather than three or four at once – you can then see which one is working. Sensible, eh?
- Look for the THR logo, which is a sign of quality.

Which herbs can help?

This table shows some commonly used herbs and what they may help with.

Herb name	Can/may help with	Caution
Agnus Castus	PMS symptoms. Hormone-regulating effect particularly useful in perimenopausal phase with fluctuating hormones.	Can interact with HRT and oral contraceptives.

Black Cohosh	Mood swings, depression, hot flushes.	Studies show mixed effectiveness.
Gingko Biloba	Circulation, therefore memory and cognitive function.	Can interfere with blood clotting – *don't* take if on warfarin or aspirin.
Sage	Hot flushes, seems to have hormone-regulatory effect.	If high blood pressure or on tamoxifen.
St John's Wort	Anxiety, depression.	Can adversely interact with many drugs.
Evening primrose oil/ starflower oil	Mood swings. Contains an essential fatty acid for breast pain and tenderness.	Aim for 240 mg daily – may interact with certain drugs.

Phytoestrogens

- Incorporating a few of these into your diet is a good idea – they occur naturally and have a weak oestrogen-like activity: flax seeds (good when shaken onto yogurt), cereals, seeds pulses, beans and vegetables.
- Diet sources: cereals, seeds pulses, beans and vegetables.

- There is growing interest and research into many countries within Asia, as they have lower rates of reported menopausal symptoms, lower cardiovascular problems, lower rates of cancers – there is a pattern occurring here even for the less observant. We can't hope to emulate the Asian diet food sources or dietary habits but we can look at our diets and add the odd supplement. They also tend to cook from fresh and take more exercise… ring a bell?!
- Phytoestrogens can be taken as a supplement, but you should not combine these with certain other supplements or HRT as they may interact. Many women opt to take a natural approach to menopause, supported through taking a phytoestrogenic supplement or holistic complimentary therapies. One recognised supplement company that has had over 15 years of scientific based research on helping women manage menopause is Promensil, who provide a range of supplements based on standardised Red Clover isoflavones, a phytoestrogen.

Vitamin D

And remember – take your *vitamin D supplement*; yes, both of you!

Alternative therapies

There may be some amongst you who think that alternative therapies are just a bit of hocus-pocus, mumbo-jumbo. That's not so – they can be incredibly useful in helping to relax and de-stress.

Pilates and yoga

The benefits of Pilates and yoga are now widely known and researched – they help with core strength, bone density, suppleness, balance, relaxation... I could go on! You should both be doing one of these on a regular basis; just go and find a class to go to and you'll see how beneficial they are.

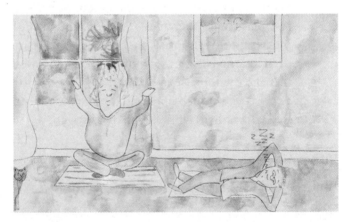

Massage

Massage offers fantastic relaxation, which is essential to every woman. You should treat her monthly – and no, a wee shoulder rub from you will not suffice!

Aromatherapy oils

Try these in bath oil form or body oils. Geranium is said to be particularly effective for menopausal symptoms.

Mindfulness and/or CBT

These are highly recommended, because developing simple coping techniques can make enormous differences not only when coping with symptoms but when coping with everyday life… and you!

Acupuncture, reflexology and hypnotherapy

These are also popular therapies – if they work then do them regularly.

Magnetic therapy

Available in the marketplace there are magnets which clip onto your pants, said to relieve menopausal symptoms. I can find no scientific research to back this up, but if it floats her boat, don't knock it!

Rest and relaxation

The most successful "alternatives" have to be simple rest and relaxation; these two things can make the most significant difference to a woman's perimenopausal transition. If you can facilitate for her to have some R&R just once or twice a week, not only will your life improve and everyone else's around you, but she will cope with her symptoms better.

POSTSCRIPT... A FINAL FEW WORDS

Well, if you've got to this page, you've either skipped the whole book – in which case, please go back and read it, as it's full of useful info – or you've gained an insight into the hormonal journey many women can be experiencing.

What about the male menopause?

Before I leave you with my final thoughts, I'll briefly direct my attention onto you, gents. There is always a debate as to whether men experience a male menopause or not. You are obviously ageing, just like she is – I know, hard to grasp but sadly true! – however, your hormones are not having such a riotous time as hers are, and are said to only decline at an average of 3% a year. Believe me, this is nothing in comparison to the female rollercoaster! However, there are some amongst you who have experienced the odd hot flush, low mood and anxiety attack, amongst other symptoms.

Whether this is down to hormones, or general ageing and pressures of life, remains to be proved one way or the other. Regardless of cause, adopting a healthy attitude to lifestyle choices will help.

I would also like to remind you that you too need to exercise your pelvic floor (yes, you do have one – what do you think is holding up all your bits and bobs?!). This will help in years to come with urinary frequency and general urinary health. It's always a good idea, too, to have a look at your own lifestyle, diet and exercise regimes. A large proportion of the male race will experience a subtle, or not so subtle, widening of their girth around middle age. This can have a knock-on effect on many health issues, including energy levels or even possibly erectile dysfunction. Now, *there's* a topic – perhaps for a follow-up book methinks…

Well, guys, I hope that, with the help of this book, your experience of it – and hers – will be easier to understand and you'll feel able to provide the support needed.

For further information on specific topics there is a blog on my website www.letstalkmenopause.co.uk and you can follow me on twitter @menopause_talk.

Good luck, everyone, look after yourselves and her – and thanks for reading!

USEFUL LINKS AND READING

Websites and links I would recommend for further reading, information and support, in alphabetical order:

Bamboo Clothing: www.bambooclothing.co.uk

Breast Cancer Care: www.breastcancercare.org.uk

British Menopause Society: wwwthebms.org.uk – excellent website particularly good to direct your primary care to – look under publications and scroll down to tools for clinicians!

British Society of Lifestyle Medicine: www.bslm.org.uk

British Heart Foundation: www.bhf.org.uk

Cognitive behavioural therapy: *Managing Hot Flushes and Night Sweats* by Myra Hunter and Melanie Smith – excellent self-help guide.

Cucumber Clothing: www.cucumberclothing.com

Daisy Network: www.daisynetwork.org.uk – essential information and support for women with premature menopause.

Drinkaware: www.drinkaware.co.uk

Dexa scan: www.nhs.uk/conditions/dexa-scan

Eve Appeal: www.eveappeal.org.uk – charity dedicated to raising awareness and funding research into the five gynaecological cancers.

Frax: www.sheffield.ac.uk/FRAX/tool.aspx

Let's Talk Menopause: www.letstalkmenopause.co.uk – useful blog posts relating to different symptoms.

Menopause Matters: www.menopausematters.co.uk – covers all aspects of the menopause and runs a very useful magazine which you can subscribe to.

Menopause Doctor: www.menopausedoctor.co.uk – covers all aspects of the menopause particularly good section on body/bio-identical hormones.

Menopause in the workplace:
www.menopauseintheworkplace.co.uk – excellent resource and support.

Nice guidelines 2015: www.nice.org.uk/guidance/NG23 – diagnosis and management of the menopause.

Osteoporosis: www.nos.org.uk

Promensil: www.promensil.co.uk – cooling spray and supplements

Southdown Duvets: southdownduvets.com

Squeezy: www.squeezyapp.co.uk – essential for pelvic floor health, men and women.

Sylk: www.sylk.co.uk

Society of Endocrinology: www.yourhormones.info

Women's Health Concern:
www.womens-health-concern.org – excellent factsheets.

All information is as accurate as possible at time of printing and is for information purposes only. It is intended for your own personal use and not intended to replace or substitute the judgment of any medical professional you may come in contact with. You should always seek advice from your healthcare professional regarding a medical condition.

ABOUT ME...

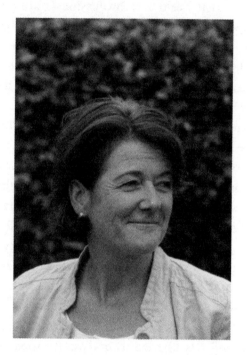

My current twitter bio sums me up really: "Bonkers about improving women's health and wellbeing specialising in the menopause. Mum of three, love cycling, netball, friends and family, tea and gin"...

I qualified as a nurse at the Edinburgh Royal Infirmary, many moons ago! After getting married and starting a family I decided to start a business following my creative interests, working as a traditional upholsterer for over 20 years, latterly incorporating a family member's fire bellows business which is still running today.

I set up Let's Talk Menopause in 2014 with the help of like-minded healthcare professionals after experiencing perimenopausal symptoms myself. The main objective being to raise awareness about the menopause, demystify it and most importantly provide easy access to information and support, whether through running workshops, through social media and on occasion contributing to programmes on BBC radio and TV. The more information everyone has, the better – women are in a better position to manage their menopause for themselves, with or without the help from health care professionals, and it helps their partners to understand more fully what they are potentially going through. The ultimate aim being a better quality of life long term, both physically and mentally for everyone.

Finally… I would just like to thank a few people… first, my fabulous family. I have an incredibly calm, and patient husband who thankfully has a brilliant sense of humour and has listened to endless menopause chat. To my wonderful three children who have had to put up with me making continual references to the menopause, but likewise are incredibly supportive and have similar senses of humour. To numerous friends who have had to listen to me rabbiting on about the menopause and what I'm up to, some who have been subjected to reading excerpts of this book – thank you for always being so supportive and for all the feedback, but, hey, a few of you are now on track to having perfect pelvic floors in later life!

A special thank you to my eldest son Harry who did the sketches throughout the book – just a bit different from his usual artwork which can be found on Instagram – Tamedartist: @_harrydevlin | tamedartist@gmail.com

And a very big thank you to Alison Jones and her team at Practical Inspiration Publishing, especially project manager Zeba, copy-editor Claire and publishing assistant Michelle, for their careful management of my work in preparation for publication.

Here's a useful checklist for you both to refer to...

Physical symptoms

Periods... that menstrual cycle

- ❑ When was your last period?

- ❑ Are your cycles regular?

- ❑ How long was your last bleed?

- ❑ Have your periods changed recently, for example... length of cycle/heaviness/flow?

- ❑ Do you take any medication or alternative remedies which help?

- ❑ Have you stopped wearing white jeans...?

_____

_____

_____

_____

_____

_____

Palpitations

- ❏ Do you ever experience palpitations?

- ❏ How severe are they?

- ❏ How long do they last for?

- ❏ How often do they occur?

- ❏ Do they accompany other symptoms?

- ❏ Is there anything you eat or drink which brings them on?

- ❏ Are there any situations that bring them on (Brad Pitt and George Clooney – or whoever floats your boat – excluded)?

- ❏ Is there anything you do which can help to reduce their intensity and frequency?

_____

_____

_____

_____

_____

_____

_____

Hot flushes/night sweats

- ❏ How often do you experience them?

- ❏ How long do they last for?

- ❏ How intense are they, on a scale of 1 to 10 (glow to dripping wet)?

- ❏ Do any foods or drinks you consume trigger them?

- ❏ Do any situations you find yourself in trigger them (back to Brad and George)?

- ❏ Do you take any medication or alternative remedies which help?

- ❏ Does anything you do help reduce the intensity and frequency of them, for example exercise or CBT?

_____

_____

_____

_____

_____

_____

Joint pains

- ❏ Do you experience aching joints?

- ❏ Which joints are affected?

- ❏ Is the pain cyclical or constant?

- ❏ Which forms of exercise help?

- ❏ Do you take medication or alternative remedies to help relieve the pain?

- ❏ Have you experienced any reduced fine motor skill ability... in other words, dropped much lately?

_____

_____

_____

_____

_____

_____

_____

_____

Headaches

- ❏ Are they cyclical or constant?

- ❏ Do they accompany other symptoms?

- ❏ Do certain foods and drinks trigger them?

- ❏ How intense are they, on a scale of 1 to 10 (muzzy to migraines)?

- ❏ Does anything you do relieve them, for example exercise or dietary intake?

- ❏ Do you take any medication or alternative remedies which help?

_____

_____

_____

_____

_____

_____

_____

_____

Insomnia

- ❏ Are your sleep patterns interrupted by other symptoms?

- ❏ Could you change your bedtime routine to help symptoms?

- ❏ Have you looked at your diet and exercise levels?

- ❏ Have you reduced any form of techy stimulation in your bedroom?

_____

_____

_____

_____

_____

_____

_____

_____

_____

Bloating and weight gain

Have you had a good look at your diet and exercise levels?

_____

_____

_____

_____

_____

_____

_____

_____

_____

_____

_____

_____

_____

Psychological symptoms

❑ Do you suffer from any of the following symptoms?

Anxiety
Poor concentration
Anger
Low mood swings
Poor memory
Irritability
Panic attacks
Lack of confidence

❑ Are the symptoms cyclical and do they accompany other symptoms?

❑ Do you currently take any medication or alternative remedies that help?

❑ Have you tried any form of alternative therapy and does it help, for example CBT?

❑ Have you looked at your diet, alcohol intake and exercise levels?

_____

_____

_____

_____

Genitourinary symptoms

❑ Do you suffer from any of the following symptoms?

Vaginal irritation
Vaginal dryness
Vaginal soreness
Vaginal discharge/infections
Urinary frequency, leakage, urgency or recurrent UTI
Reduced sex drive/libido
Uncomfortable/painful sexual intercourse

❑ Do you currently take any medication or alternative remedies that help?

❑ Do you do your pelvic floor exercises?

❑ Have you downloaded the Squeezy app?

_____

_____

_____

_____

_____

_____

Lifestyle diet and exercise

❑ Do you regularly exercise every week?

❑ How many times?

❑ Do you do a variety of exercise, including aerobic and pilates/yoga?

❑ If exercise doesn't float your boat, you really need to do some... have you tried HIIT... we are talking ten minutes a day?

❑ Do you eat a healthy, balanced diet?

❑ Do you eat regular meals?

❑ Do you drink plenty of water?

❑ What is your weekly alcohol intake? Come on, be honest!

❑ Do you smoke?

❑ Have you tried any alternative therapies like reflexology or CBT?

❑ Do you take any alternative remedies or supplements?

❑ Note down any medication and alternatives you are on.

_____

_____